Weight Loss

Diet Cookbook And Weight Loss Motivation Tips For Creating New Habits To Lose Body & Belly Fat, And Living A Healthier And Happier Life!

Chris Smith

Copyright © 2015 Chris Smith

STOP!!! Before you read any further....Would you like to know the Secrets of Body Transformation?

If your answer is yes, then you are not alone. Thousands of people are looking for the secret to rapidly burn body fat, keep the weight off, become healthier, and truly transform their body and life for good.

If you have been searching for these answers without much luck, you are in the right place!

Not only will you gain incredible insight in this book, but because I want to make sure to give you as much value as possible, right now for a limited time you can get full **100% FREE access to a VIP bonus EBook** entitled **THE 7 KEYS TO BODY TRANSFORMATION!**

Just Go Here For Free Instant Access:

www.liveFitVIP.com

Legal Notice

Disclaimer Notice

Table Of Contents

Introduction

I want to thank you and congratulate you for purchasing the book, *Weight Loss: Diet Cookbook And Weight Loss Motivation Tips For Creating New Habits To Lose Body & Belly Fat, And Living A Healthier And Happier Life!*

This "Weight Loss" book contains tips, strategies, and recipes that will help you lose weight. The book is divided into different chapters for you to easily follow and digest the information. The book provides basic information, as well as clearing up misconceptions about the presented topics to give you the best insight regarding weight loss.

Thanks again for purchasing this book, I hope you enjoy it!

Chapter 1: Overview Of Weight Loss

If you want to lose weight, then you have to watch your lifestyle. Particularly, your focus is on diet and exercise. Both are equally important in achieving your desired weight. However, as you might have predicted from the title, this book will deal with the diet part.

To lose weight, you have to consume fewer calories than what you burn. Your consumed calories will be stored as fat if not burned. Your diet is where your calorie intake comes from. Your exercise or workout takes care of burning calories. Thus, it is important to plan your diet. You have to be closely aware of your macronutrient intake. The three macronutrients are carbohydrates, fat and protein.

Carbohydrates

Weight loss advocates view carbohydrates, shortened as "carbs", as a black sheep or a mortal enemy. This is evident on how much "low-carb diets" are popular today. However, it is one of the most important components of your diet. It is your body's main source of energy after all. When you consume carbs, the body converts it to glucose that is used by your cells, including those of the muscles and the brain, as fuel. The point is that you shouldn't completely remove carbs from your diet. However, it is perhaps the most important macronutrient to watch in your diet.

Basically, your carb consumption must match your level of physical activity. However, it's not all about the quantity. You must also be aware of the quality. Simply cutting down on carb consumption won't make you lose weight effectively. Experts divide carbs into good and bad ones. Discussing the details of what makes a carb good or bad will be lengthy. It is worth a whole other article (or even a whole book). For our purposes, you just need to know which ones are good sources of carbs for your diet and which ones to avoid.

Fruits and vegetables are good sources of carbs. The carbs they provide are good and they contain high levels of vitamins and minerals to keep you healthy. Furthermore, they are high in fiber which contributes to healthy bowel movement and makes you feel full faster (i.e. aids in preventing you from overeating).

On the other hand, you must minimize your consumption of chocolates, cakes, candies, and other types of sweets. They are high in sugar and calories that significantly contribute to tooth decay and unhealthy weight gain. The same is true for soft drinks.

Fats

Fat, like carbs, provide energy. However, they are harder to break down. Thus, the body only uses them as a secondary source if you run out of carbs. Before the discovery of carbs as the antagonist of weight loss, it was fat that held that connotation. That belief has long been debunked. Fats are also a necessary part of diet. Like in the case of carbs, it is also not just about the amount, but the kind of fat you consume. Not all fats are created equal. There are also good and bad fat.

Saturated fats and trans fats are bad fat. These fats cause weight gain. Furthermore, they contribute to increase in your body's cholesterol levels and clogging of arteries, which lead to higher risk of cardiovascular diseases.

On the other hand, omega-3s and unsaturated fats (both poly- and mono-) are good fats. They have the opposite effects of bad fats. They are good for the heart and have some other benefits such as helping in mood management, weight control and fighting fatigue.

Protein

Protein is essential in the diet and not as troublesome to watch as the carbs and fats. The body needs protein for tissue repair, growth (especially for pregnant women, children, and teens), immunity, hormone and enzyme production, muscle buildup, and alternative energy source.

Scientific research shows that aside from the functions mentioned above, protein helps in weight loss. This is by heightening the metabolic rate (i.e. helps burn more calories) and making you feel full faster (i.e. reducing calorie intake).

When you eat protein-rich foods, it contributes to weight gain, but the weight you gain is muscle not fat. That means healthy weight gain. The right amount of protein for a person depends on several factors, namely, age, height, current physique, and physical activity level. As a quick reference, here are some amounts:

- Adult male with average build and sedentary lifestyle: 56 grams
- Adult female with average build and sedentary lifestyle: 46 grams

These amounts are just minimum values to avoid protein deficiency. You'll have to consume more if you aim to build muscles.

Too much of anything is bad. Protein is not an exception. There is a possibility to overeat protein. While it is not as easy to consume too much protein compared to carbs and fat, excessive protein will cause unpleasant things to your body:

- If coupled with lower amounts of other macronutrient intake, the body will turn the excess protein into calories. It wouldn't be turned into muscle, but fat which is a weight gain you don't want.
- If you don't couple high protein intake with enough water, you will be prone to dehydration.
- Too much protein may also cause intestinal irritation.

There are good and bad sources of protein, just like with fat and carbs. However, protein sources should not be simply labeled as "good" or "bad" since some protein sources that have been labeled as "bad" are actually not bad – as long as you keep them in moderation (unlike with the bad carbs and fat that you should totally avoid). There are other factors as to why you should be careful. So, you should just know what to watch. Here are some reminders regarding common protein sources:

- While providing good amounts of protein, red meat contains saturated fat. It's a good practice to limit your intake of red meat, especially processed ones (e.g. bacon, hotdog, deli meats, and sausage).
- With chicken, there is not much worry since it is white meat. What you should do is to be aware of the parts you eat. Chicken breasts are good. Remember also that it is recommended to stray away from the skin because of its fat content. The same is true for turkey.

On the other hand, here are some recommendations:

- Opt for lean meat as much as possible. A good meat shop categorizes lean cut meats.
- White meat is nice as it contains low fat.
- Fish is also a good source, particularly salmon. Aside from good amount of proteins, it also contains the healthy omega-3s.
- You can also get protein from plant sources – soy products, whole grains, beans, seeds and nuts. As a bonus, you get a good dose of fiber and unsaturated fat.

Being familiar with the macronutrients will contribute greatly with your weight loss goals.

Chapter 2: Low Carb Diets – How Do They Work?

As discussed in the previous chapter, watching carbs in your diet would do wonders for weight loss. You're probably aware of the popularity of low-carb diets nowadays. The good news is that they indeed work. However, you should not just follow any low-carb diet you find out there – not all of them are created equal. If done wrong, you might compromise your health. The best course of action is to consult with an expert dietician or nutritionist.

In a low-carb diet, you restrict your carbohydrate intake while increasing your protein and fat intake. However, it is not only about restricting your amounts. You have to carefully choose the sources of your carb, protein and fat intake. You've seen the good and bad sources of these macronutrients in the previous chapter.

When you follow a good low-carb diet properly, you can lose weight. However, the benefits are beyond that. It can also prevent certain health conditions including diabetes, hypertension, metabolic syndrome and cardiovascular disease. If you are already suffering from these, then a low-carb diet can help improve them.

As with all things, there are right and wrong ways to do low-carb diets. Sometimes, when people get desperate about losing weight, they cut down calories too drastically. They may fall into eating disorders. There can be many other risks such as headache, fatigue, diarrhea or constipation, weakness and even bad breath. Also, too much restriction in carb intake may lead to nutritional deficiencies, chronic diseases, gastrointestinal disturbances and bone loss.

Chapter 3: Motivation Tips For Creating New Habits To Lose Weight

During your quest for weight loss, you'll face many obstacles. You'll be changing habits that we all know is not easy. Your biggest opponent will be yourself. That's why it's important to keep your motivation strong. As you might have figured out from the title, this chapter is about motivation tips for weight loss diet.

Set Realistic Goals

The first step is setting your goals. In this stage, it is important that you set realistic goals. Your goals should be just enough to challenge you. If it's too easy, then you won't be motivated to put effort. Attaining each would not mean much to you. On the other hand, if it's too hard, you're simply setting up yourself for failure. You'll be disappointed and likely won't keep your diet up.

Your goals must be focused and specific. Set smaller benchmarks. For example, lose 5 pounds in a month or go down by one dress size – such are realistically attainable and are more likely to boost your confidence.

Take it Slow

Next tip is to take things slowly. Dieting for weight loss requires lifestyle changes and such things take time. Make changes little by little. You can handle them more easily. If you make drastic changes, then you'll shock your system. Starvation is one of the greatest enemies of people who are trying to lose weight. Your body has the instinct to eat until you're full and instincts are hard to fight off head on.

For example, if you cut off 1000 calories from your usual diet right off the bat, you'll feel hungry. Your body will send off hunger pangs stronger than ever. You'll feel frustrated and irritated. These kinds of emotion will most likely make you give up. Instead, start with around a 200-calorie reduction. This way, your body won't feel it that much. Keep in mind: optimal levels of weight loss are around 1-2 pounds a week. You'll avoid frustration and, as a result, you'll be able to stay on your diet.

Expect Setbacks

When on a weight loss diet, expect to encounter setbacks. Even the hardiest people are prone to surrender to temptations once in a while. If you do this, don't be too hard on yourself. That's because the tendency is for you to think, "Oh, I already blew. I just can't do this." Then, you'll just give up altogether.

Trash the Perfectionist Mindset

The next one is related to the previous tip. That is to not be a perfectionist. There is perhaps no hindrance to success more powerful than a perfectionist thinking. You'd view your small slips as catastrophic failure. This fuels frustration and we already know what frustration does. So what if you indulge in sweets once? You recognize that you slip up. That is something you shouldn't do, but don't wallow in it. Forget about it and move on. You can use tomorrow to eat healthier.

Buddy System

Do things with a buddy. You can definitely find someone who shares the same goal as yours. With a buddy, you have someone to talk to about your goals, dietary measures, daily progress, and most importantly, frustrations. This will help you feel better and renew your motivation. You can remind each other about your goals and stuff.

Be Patient

Patience – you'll need lots and lots of it. In weight loss dieting, there is something called "weight loss plateau." You're doing your diet properly and coupling it with adequate exercise. You're not even slipping up. You check the scales every day and the numbers are steadily decreasing. Then, one day, the number stays on one spot for some consecutive days. You've just hit the plateau. According to experts, this is just a normal stage in the process of weight loss. Instead of thinking that you're doing something wrong, think about the progress you've made so far and pat yourself on the back (figuratively, of course).

You might want to try something different when you hit this stage. Maybe cut a further 50 calories from your diet or add a 20-minute walk to your daily exercise. This can be the jumpstart you need to get over that plateau.

Reward Yourself

Give yourself a reward for your benchmarks. In the first part, you have set these. Once you attain them, give yourself something good. Anything that makes you happy will do – as long as it's not food, of course. Buy a new shirt to celebrate your new size, play your favorite game, or get a massage. Celebrating these benchmarks will reinforce your resolve.

Plan Your Maintenance

Last but not the least is planning your maintenance. In many cases, it will be easier to strip weight than keep it off. This happens because of a wrong mindset. You have to view healthy eating as a life goal instead of a one-time project. Otherwise, you'll be eating unhealthy once you reach your desired weight and before you know it, you're gaining it back. So, form your maintenance plan early.

It is recommended to consult with an expert in forming your plan. This is a good way to maximize the effectiveness of the plan. You can consult a nutritionist, a health counselor, a dietician, or a trainer for this. Couple it with making an exercise plan with the help of an expert (e.g. gym instructor or fitness coach) as well. The help of an expert is valuable in starting your plan right and determining exactly what you need, so that you can more easily maintain your healthy eating and exercise habits beyond the time you reached your ideal weight.

Chapter 4: Clean Eating And Weight Loss

In trying to lose weight, one of the things that people do is clean eating. Advocates of clean eating say that it has great promises to health, especially for weight loss. Some will even claim that you will no longer need to count your calorie intake if you eat clean.

There are several promises of clean eating. You'll lose an average of 3 pounds a week. Beyond that, you also become healthier. You have more energy. You'll have glowing skin. You'll have bright and alert eyes. You'll have strong teeth and gums. You also won't feel starved. You get all these without the need to count calories? Good, right?

Clean eating is a good habit to incorporate in your weight loss plan. It is more than recommended. However, it is still best to track the quantity of your macronutrient intake.

What is it?

Well, what exactly is "clean eating"?

Clean eating is a lifestyle that is composed of several principles. They are as follows:

- Each day, you eat six (6) small meals.
- You must not skip breakfast and have it within one hour of getting up.
- Lean protein and complex carbohydrates must be part of each meal.
- Consume two to three servings of good fats each day.
- Eat fruits and vegetables to get vitamins, minerals, fiber, and enzymes.
- Have complete control of your portions.
- Drink lots of water – 2 to 3 liters each day.

In clean eating, there are certain foods to avoid:

- Foods that are over-processed, particularly white sugar and flour
- Artificial sweeteners
- Beverages with high sugar content, like juice and soda

- Alcohol
- Foods containing chemical additives, such as sodium nitrate and food dyes
- Saturated and trans fats
- Foods containing preservatives
- Artificial food, like processed cheese slices
- Anti-foods – these are the ones with high calorie density but doesn't have nutritional value

That's clean eating. The question now is, "Does it fulfill its promises?" Well, with principles like that, it's not hard to see why eating clean should work. It follows the recommendations of a healthy lifestyle and such an eating habit will help greatly in weight loss.

However, some clean eating programs out there recommend supplements that medical experts aren't too fond of. Having that awareness is important. Also, like mentioned before, some will say that you no longer need to count calories. That's not entirely true. Counting your calories and macronutrient intake is a good practice to discipline your dietary habits.

Chapter 5: Herbal Remedies For Weight Loss

In the previous chapters, you've learned to be wary of processed food. It is indeed seen as one of the leading causes of obesity. In the past, our ancestors didn't have the obesity problem because of their physically active lifestyle and their foods are all natural. So, when it comes to losing weight, going all-natural is one of the recommended practices.

To aid in weight loss, some people use herbal remedies. Here are some of those remedies:

- Green Tea. It is known for its high antioxidant content, but green tea also promotes weight loss. This is because of its thermogenic properties. Thermogenesis is basically the heat production process of organisms. This process helps in burning energy and oxidizing fat. Furthermore, green tea has a good satiation rate, meaning it helps you feel full faster so you don't eat more than necessary. Green tea also helps in reducing the fat your body absorbs from food. This helps not only in losing weight, but also in reducing your body's cholesterol levels.

- Ginseng. Chinese people have used ginseng since long ago. It serves as medicine for stamina, energy, and general health. In recent times, scientists have discovered that ginseng has abilities that help in controlling diabetes and losing weight. One of these abilities is the reduction of the cells' capability to store fat. As such, ginseng helps you lose weight by making your body store less fat and giving you energy that will keep you active (i.e. making you spend more calories).

- Hibiscus. The flowers of this herb contain lots of minerals, flavonoids, and other nutrients. For one, it has amylase inhibitors that lower your body's fat and carb absorption. Hibiscus breaks them down so your body can expel them, instead of being absorbed. Moreover, it has diuretic properties that aid in shedding water weight.

- Pu-erh Tea. This herb was first cultivated in Pu-erh village in China, hence the name, around 2000 years ago. This particularly enhances the function of your spleen, making it easier for your body to absorb nutrients from food and expel excess fluid. It also heightens your metabolism so you burn fat – faster and in more amounts.

- Kelp. This is an extensive part of Japanese diet. It won't be surprising if it's one of the reasons they are relatively slimmer. Kelp is a good source of iodine, which stimulates the thyroid gland. Thus, your metabolism is always on a good rate. Then, it also has alginate, a compound that has been shown by research to reduce fat absorption.

- Coleus forskohlii. This herb native to the southern parts of Asia is a member of the mint family. It is also called Indian coleus. The roots of this herb contain forskolin, a compound that incites the thyroid gland.

- Guggul Herb. Since ancient times, this herb has been used for medicinal purposes. Now, modern studies have backed up its weight loss capabilities. Guggul extract contains guggulsterone, which helps in keeping your metabolic rate at optimal levels.

- Yerba Mate. This traditional drink in South America is widely known as tea, but it is actually more similar to coffee. It contains caffeine that gives you stamina, but Yerba Mate also increases your calorie burning rate.

- Grapefruit. This contains Naringenin, a flavonoid that has been found to aid in balancing sugar levels in the blood and keep metabolic syndrome at bay. Metabolic syndrome can make you gain weight and may cause diabetes.

- Prickly Pear. This cactus plant has been used as traditional medicine for high cholesterol, diabetes, and even obesity. Also called Indian fig, the fruit of this plant is high in antioxidants. It helps control blood sugar levels that in turn lowers bad cholesterol levels and helps in weight loss.

- Gurmar. The leaves of this plant have been in use for a long time in treating several diseases including kidney stones, liver and spleen enlargement, obesity, and diabetes. This herb reduces your cravings for sweets, which will aid in controlling your weight.

These herbal remedies are good. Remember, though, that it's best to consult a medical expert before taking them. This is mandatory if you are already under medication (e.g. for diabetes).

Chapter 6: Coconut Oil For Weight Loss

Another thing that has been claimed to aid in weight loss is coconut oil, particularly virgin coconut oil. This claim is backed up by scientific research. So, you can incorporate it in your quest for weight loss if you want.

How does coconut oil aid in weight loss? There are several ways.

Coconut oil contains medium chain triglycerides. Now, we won't be going through a whole chemistry lesson here to explain that. What's important to know is that they are processed differently by the digestive system. They go straight to your liver and are used right away.

Coconut oil enhances metabolism and increases the calories you burn even at rest. Coconut oil has thermo-genic properties, meaning the calories you get from it increase the amount of energy you burn compared to the same amount of calories from other fat sources.

Coconut oil helps reduce your appetite. Thus, you eat less without even thinking about it. The medium chain triglycerides in coconut oil make you feel full faster and so, your calorie intake is reduced.

Coconut oil helps you reduce visceral fat. The body stores fat in two ways. Fat under your skin is called subcutaneous fat. Fat that surround your organs in the belly is called visceral fat. Visceral fat is the more dangerous of the two. Several studies have shown that while coconut oil does not cause overnight fat reduction, it does cause long-term reduction of visceral fat.

With these benefits, you can lose weight by using coconut oil for cooking from now on. Some people actually consume a few teaspoons of virgin coconut oil a day by itself.

Chapter 7: Alkaline Weight Loss Tips

Another weigh loss thing out there is the alkaline diet. Also called "alkaline ash diet" or "alkaline acid diet" by some, it is a diet that is promoted foremost for aiding weight loss, but is also reported to have other benefits such as decreasing the likelihood of arthritis or cancer.

The idea behind this kind of diet is that many foods, especially processed ones cause your body to produce acids that have bad effects on the human body. So, if you choose foods that cause your body to be more alkaline, you will be healthier. You will lose weight and protect yourself from certain conditions.

Well, does it work? Well, yes. It can work but not for the advertised explanation you see above.

The alkaline diet is supposed to keep the pH level (the value which determines how acidic or alkaline something is) of your blood in check. However, what you eat doesn't have a significant effect on your blood's pH level. Your body actually has mechanisms to keep it constant.

However, the alkaline diet may indeed have benefits. You lose weight and become healthier because the recommended foods on an alkaline diet are healthy foods. You eat more fruits and vegetables and consume a lot of water. Furthermore, the alkaline diet tells you to stray away from alcohol, caffeine, and processed food. As you might have realized, it aligns with the principles of clean eating.

So, following tips from the alkaline diet concept can also help you lose weight. Here are some of them.

- Drink a lot of water. Keeping yourself properly hydrated is important to overall health.
- Avoid foods that contain food dyes, additives, and preservatives.
- Stay away from artificial sweeteners.
- Avoid stress and/or learn better handling of it.

- Breathe properly. Many of us don't breath properly without realizing it. Proper breathing lets your lungs work to its full capacity. Use your diaphragm and fill the bottom of your lungs first. Take several deep breaths a day.
- Keep your fridge stocked with ready-to-cook vegetables.

Chapter 8: Tips For Getting Into Shape And Living A Healthier, Happier Life

In your quest for changing your diet for weight loss, you will find that whichever methods you choose, they will be more effective if you follow these tips for getting in shape and generally living a healthier life:

- It's better to exercise daily. You'll lose weight if you burn more calories than what you consume. So, it's possible to lose weight by just reducing your calorie consumption based on your current level of physical activity. However, it's better to add daily exercise to increase your physical activity. This way, you can give allowance to the restrictions you will make in your calorie intake.

- Don't make your exercises longer, increase the intensity instead. Exercising for longer takes up your time, which you could have used for your hobbies or something productive. Besides, exercising for longer than 90 minutes can actually affect your body negatively, working against your goals.

- Keep yourself positive. This does not only help you keep stress at bay, but will also help keep you motivated in staying with your healthy life habits. You feel happier overall and such will do wonders for your body. Remember that positive thinking is not disregarding negative outcomes – it's about facing them with the right attitude if they do happen.

- Start slow. You never need to be harsh on yourself. Push yourself little by little. Healthy living is not a race, it's a marathon. If you see others accomplishing things fast, you don't need to compare your progress with them. Your circumstances are likely different from theirs. Do not compete with others. Instead, concentrate on being better than yourself yesterday.

- Tell the people you care about of your health goals. They will support you, which will help you keep a positive perspective on the things you're doing.

- Consistency is the key. As mentioned before, healthy living is not a one-time project – it's a lifestyle. Commit yourself into maintaining your healthy habits and avoid coming back to your old ways.

- Be an advocate. Use your progress and experience in healthy living to inspire others. Give advice, but don't be pushy. If you are helping others achieve what you have achieved, you will also find more reasons to keep yourself healthy.

Chapter 9: Simple Recipes For Weight Loss

You have learned many tips and information about weight loss. To help you further, here are simple recipes you can incorporate in your diet plans.

Breakfasts

1.   Eggs and Greens

Heat a skillet and put in half a tablespoon of olive oil. Sauté 2 cups of spinach and 1 cup of sliced mushrooms and put them on a plate. Add another half tablespoon of olive oil to the skillet and cook the egg (recommended: sunny side-up). Add the egg to the veggies and add some chili sauce if desired.

2.   Home Fries and Sausage

Heat the sausage. Cube 1 sweet potato. Sauté the potato cubes and 1 cup of kale in a separate pan. Sprinkle red pepper flakes when done.

3.   Savory English Muffin

Cut one English muffin in half. Put the ham, cheese, and kale on top of the halves. Sprinkle a bit of olive oil. Toast in the oven for 10 minutes at 375 degrees Fahrenheit.

4.   Smoked Salmon Toast

Spread 1 ½ tablespoons of cream cheese on the bread. Layer the salmon, onions, and chives.

5.   Waffles with Maple Syrup and Blueberries

Put 1/3 cup of frozen blueberries and two teaspoons of maple syrup together and microwave them for 2 to 3 minutes or until berries get thawed. Toast the waffles. Top with the still warm syrup mix and sprinkle with a tablespoon of pecans.

6.   Bacon and Spinach Omelet

Put in 1 egg, 2 egg whites, crumbled two slices of bacon, and 1 cup spinach together and whisk them. Heat a skillet and coat with cooking spray. Cook the mixture. Serve with butter and toasted bread.

7. Pumpkin and Granola Parfait

Mix together 6 ounces of low-fat yogurt, two teaspoons of honey, and ¼ teaspoon of pumpkin-pie spice. Crumble 1 bar of whole-grain granola bar. Layer the yogurt mixture, crumbled granola, and half cup of canned pumpkin in a bowl.

8. Bagel with Cream Cheese and Tomato

Cut a small whole-grain bagel in half and toast them. Spread cream cheese on them (around a tablespoon for each half). Top each with a large slice of tomato. Add salt and pepper if desired.

9. Pancakes with Peanut Butter and Banana

Chop half a small banana. Mix it and 2 teaspoons of peanut butter with 1/3 cup of whole-grain pancake batter (prepared beforehand). Cook the pancakes and top with honey (1 teaspoon).

10. Vanilla Spice Apple French Toast

Whisk together 1 egg, two egg whites, cinnamon, and nutmeg. Dip two slices of whole-grain bread into the egg mixture. Sauté each bread thoroughly. Top with slices of apple.

Lunch

11. Baja Chicken Bowl

Heat a skillet. Put in 1 teaspoon olive oil. Sauté half a cup of thin slices of red bell pepper, ¼ cup of frozen corn, ¼ cup of black beans, and 2 ounces of cooked chicken (diced). Serve with half cup of cooked brown rice. Add some salsa.

12. Spicy Thai Noodles with Tofu

Cook whole grain spaghetti noodles (2 ounces). Heat a teaspoon of sesame oil in a skillet. Put in 1 teaspoon of honey and 1 teaspoon of hot chili sauce. Once hot, add 2 ounces of tofu (cubed) and 2 cups of broccoli slaw. Sauté the mixture for 5 minutes. Add the cooked spaghetti and toss. Sprinkle 1 tablespoon of crumbled peanuts, a tablespoon of cilantro leaves, and thin slices of scallion.

13. Greek Salad with Tuna

•   Get a large bowl. Mix together 2 teaspoons of olive oil, 2 teaspoons of red wine vinegar, half a teaspoon of dried oregano, and a pinch of salt and pepper. Whisk them. Add in 3 cups of romaine (chopped), 2 ½ ounces of tune (water-packed), half cup of cucumber (diced), half cup of tomato (diced), half cup whole-grain couscous (cooked), a tablespoon of feta (crumbled), and Kalamata olives (4 pieces, chopped). Toss the ingredients together.

14. Crab-Quinoa Salad

•   Toss together 1 tablespoon of grapefruit juice, 2 teaspoons of olive oil, 1 teaspoon mustard, and a pinch of salt and pepper in a bowl. Add quinoa (1/2 cup, cooked and cooled), crab meat (2 ounces), and avocado (1/4, chopped). Toss and serve with salad greens.

15. Artichoke, Chicken and Spinach Panino

Top a slice of whole grain bread with baby spinach (1/2 cup), artichoke hearts (1/4 cup, quartered), chicken breast slices (2 ½ ounces), and provolone (1 slice). Cover with another slice of bread. Grill each side.

16. Pita Pockets of Turkey, Apple, and Cheese

•   Divide 1 whole wheat Pita pocket in half. Stuff each half with turkey breasts (1 ounce, sliced), apple (1/4, thinly sliced), and baby spinach (1/2 cup). Serve with another apple half.

17. Pesto Pizza with White Beans and Roasted Red Peppers

Preheat a broiler. Spread pesto (1 tablespoon) on a large whole-grain pita. Place it on a baking sheet. Top it with white beans (1/2 cup) and roasted red peppers (1/2 cup, chopped). Sprinkle with Parmesan (1 tablespoon, grated). Broil for 5 minutes.

18. Quinoa Edamame Salad

Cook dry quinoa (1/4 cup) in a pot with around a cup of water until consistency becomes like rice. In a separate pan, pour 2-3 cups of vegetable broth. Let it simmer. Add onions (1/3 cup, chopped), tomatoes (8-10 pieces, small, sliced in half), and edamame (1 cup, shelled). Transfer the quinoa to a heated pan. Stir-fry it. Add squeezed lemons, mustard, and agave nectar as dressing.

Conclusion

Thank you again for purchasing this book on *Weight Loss: Diet Cookbook And Weight Loss Motivation Tips For Creating New Habits To Lose Body & Belly Fat, And Living A Healthier And Happier Life!*

I am extremely excited to pass this information along to you, and I am so happy that you now have read and can hopefully implement these strategies going forward.

I hope this book was able to help you understand the importance of diet in losing weight and how to apply the tips and information presented here to form your own weight loss plans.

The next step is to get started using this information and to hopefully live a healthier and happier life!

Please don't be someone who just reads this information and doesn't apply it, the strategies in this book will only benefit you if you use them!

If you know of anyone else that could benefit from the information presented here please inform them of this book.

Finally, if you enjoyed this book and feel it has added value to your life in any way, please take the time to share your thoughts and post a review on Amazon. It'd be greatly appreciated!

Thank you and good luck!

Preview Of:

Low Carb Diet

The Best Guide To Low Carb - Lose Fat And Get A Fast Metabolism In 7 Days With This Weight Loss Blood Sugar Solution Diet!

Introduction

I want to thank you and congratulate you for purchasing the book, *"Low Carb Diet: The Best Guide To Low Carb - Lose Fat And Get A Fast Metabolism In 7 Days With This Weight Loss Blood Sugar Solution Diet!"*.

This book contains proven steps and strategies on how to get the body of your dreams!

Don't let another week pass you by living life out of shape! The extra weight around your waistline or hips is more than just a problem of how you look in the mirror. Especially if it is not burned off in the near future, it can cause a host of other problems relating to your health and longevity. You owe it to yourself and the ones close to you to get in the best shape of your life.

Imagine how nice it would feel to look in the mirror and be happy with what you see on the outside and be comforted knowing that you are much healthier on the inside.

If you are serious about finally losing weight and keeping it off, then you have come to the right place. "Low Carb Diet: Low Carb Diet Solution - In as Little as 7 Days You Can Lose Weight Fast Using This Low Carb Diet Plan!" is the solution you have been looking for that allows you to literally create the body of your dreams, and what's even better is you will start seeing results within the first 7 days. Anyone who truly wants to lose weight can use these principles and be on their way in a matter of days! Don't waste another week, begin living life to the fullest today!

This book does not offer a drastic solution. But it will show you how to customize your low carb meals for seven days so you can start experiencing your desired weight loss results.

Thanks again for purchasing this book, I hope you enjoy it!

Chapter 1 – What Is A Low Carb Diet?

I am so excited for you! If you are reading this far, it means that you truly are looking for change in your life! You are tired of not living to your full potential, and ready to start living the way you were intended to. That's great, and what better way to start than by creating the best body of your life!

Keep that enthusiasm high because that is exactly what will carry you through to reaching your goals. The truth is the most important factor in your goals being obtained is you. You are the one that must "decide". You must simply make a choice that no matter what, you will reach your goal. If you simply do this, than I am confident you will succeed.

So let's get started! But Before we jump straight into what you should eat and the details of the diet, we need to make sure you are caught up to speed on the basics of a low carb diet.

If you've been dieting or have at least tried to do something about your weight, then you might have heard or read about low carb diets. Some of the popular fad-diets that can be classified as low carb diets include Sugar Busters Diet, the well-known South Beach Diet, the ever popular Zone Diet, Atkins, and pretty much every other diet you may have heard of.

As you should know by now, the term "low carb diet" has actually been applied to many different diets. It's a really broad classification of different diets that limit carbohydrate intake. Some people call them low glycemic diets while others refer to them as reduced carbohydrate diets.

The common denominator for these diets that belong to the "low carb" class is that they require, just as the name suggests, a diet that excludes foods that are heavy in carbohydrates. These are foods that are referred to as glycemic. There are lists of foods and their glycemic index to guide people going on any low carb diet.

So How Low Carb is Low Carb, Really?

You may consult your doctor about how low carb your diet should be; this is the smartest thing you should do before engaging in any diet. The dietary guidelines in the United States state that around 50 to 65 percent of a person's calorie intake for any given day should come from carbs.

Generally speaking, you should simply have less than 50% to 65% calories coming from carbohydrate sources of any variant in your daily diet. There are low carb diets that recommend only 20% or less of your daily caloric intake. If you want to live off a low carb diet for weight loss, keeping your carbohydrate intake to less than 20% of your daily caloric requirement is advised. Of course, you should make sure that you substitute this with another calorie source, mostly vegetables. With this kind of drastic drop in carbohydrate consumption, not all people are able to handle the dietary changes.

Your body will react. You can feel uneasy because of cravings for the carbs that you are used to having. That is why you will have to slowly adjust your carb intake up to the point when your body can take the loss of carbs. You may think that's a bit of a hit and miss approach, but the fact remains that everyone has a different tolerance for carb loss.

Thanks for Previewing My Exciting Book Entitled:

"Low Carb Diet: The Best Guide To Low Carb - Lose Fat And Get A Fast Metabolism In 7 Days With This Weight Loss Blood Sugar Solution Diet!"

To purchase this book, simply go to the Amazon Kindle store and simply search:

"LOW CARB DIET"

Then just scroll down until you see my book. You will know it is mine because you will see my name "Chris Smith" underneath the title.

Alternatively, you can visit my author page on Amazon to see this book and other work I have done. Thanks so much, and please don't forget your free bonuses

DON'T LEAVE YET! - CHECK OUT YOUR FREE BONUSES BELOW!

Free Bonus Offer: Get Free Access To The www.LiveFitVIP.com VIP Newsletter!

Once you enter your email address you will immediately get free access to this awesome newsletter!

But wait, right now if you join now for free you will also get free access to the "The 7 Keys To Body Transformation" free EBook!

To claim both your FREE VIP NEWSLETTER MEMBERSHIP and your FREE BONUS Ebook on THE 7 KEYS TO BODY TRANSFORMATION!

Just Go To:

www.liveFitVIP.com